The Definitive K
Cookbook Recipes ᵢₒᵢ ᴅ._ᵤ

Delicious and Healthy Recipes to Improve and Boost Your Metabolism

Veronica Lang

Table of contents

Chocolate Peanut Butter Chaffle

Servings: 2

Prep time: 5 min. Cook time: 10 min **Ingredients:**

½ cup shredded mozzarella cheese 1 Tbsp cocoa powder

1 Tbsp powdered sweetener 2 Tbsp peanut butter

½ tsp vanilla 1 egg

2 Tbsp crushed peanuts 2 Tbsp whipped cream

¼ cup sugar-free chocolate syrup

Directions:

1 Combine mozzarella, egg, vanilla, peanut butter, cocoa powder, and sweetener in a bowl. Add in peanuts and mix well.

2 Turn on waffle maker and oil it with cooking spray.

3 Pour one half of the batter into waffle maker, cook for 4 minutes, and then transfer to a plate. Top with whipped cream, peanuts, and sugar-free chocolate syrup.

Nutrition Value per Servings:

Carbs - 6 G Fat - 17 G Protein - 15 G Calories – 236

Pumpkin Pecan Chaffles

Servings: 2

Prep time: 10 min. Cook time: 10 min. **Ingredients:**

1 egg

½ cup mozzarella cheese grated 1 Tbsp pumpkin puree

½ tsp pumpkin spice

1 tsp erythritol low carb sweetener 2 Tbsp almond flour

2 Tbsp pecans, toasted chopped 1 cup heavy whipped cream

¼ cup low carb caramel sauce

Directions:

1 Turn on waffle maker to heat and oil it with cooking spray. In a bowl, beat egg.

2 Mix in mozzarella, pumpkin, flour, pumpkin spice, and erythritol. Stir in pecan pieces.

3 Spoon one half of the batter into waffle maker and spread evenly. Close and cook for 5 minutes.

4 Remove cooked waffles to a plate. Repeat with remaining batter. Serve with pecans, whipped cream, and low carb caramel sauce.

Nutrition Value per Servings:

Carbs - 4 G Fat - 17 G Protein - 11 G Calories – 210

Italian Cream Chaffle Sandwich-Cake

Ingredients:

4 oz cream cheese, softened, at room tempereture 4 eggs

1 Tbsp melted butter 1 tsp vanilla extract

½ tsp cinnamon

1 Tbsp monk fruit sweetener 4 Tbsp coconut flour

1 Tbsp almond flour

1½ teaspoons baking powder

1 Tbsp coconut, shredded and unsweetened 1 Tbsp walnuts, chopped

FOR THE ITALIAN CREAM FROSTING:

2 oz cream cheese, softened, at room temperature 2 Tbsp butter room temp

2 Tbsp monk fruit sweetener ½ tsp vanilla

Directions:

1 Combine cream cheese, eggs, melted butter, vanilla, sweetener, flours, and baking powder in a blender. Add walnuts and coconut to the mixture.

2 Blend to get a creamy mixture.

3 Turn on waffle maker to heat and oil it with cooking
spray.

4 Add enough batter to fill waffle maker. Cook for 2-3
minutes, until chaffles are done. Remove and let them
cool.

5 Mix all frosting ingredients in another bowl. Stir until
smooth and creamy. Frost the chaffles once they have
cooled.

6 Top with cream and more nuts
Nutrition Value per Servings:Carbs - 31 G Fat - 2 G
Protein - 5 G Calories – 168

Chocolate Cherry Chaffles

Servings: 1

Prep time: 5 min. Cook time: 5 min. **Ingredients:**

1 Tbsp almond flour 1 Tbsp cocoa powder

1 Tbsp sugar free sweetener ½ tsp baking powder 1 whole egg

½ cup mozzarella cheese shredded

2 Tbsp heavy whipping cream whipped 2 Tbsp sugar free cherry
   pie filling

1 Tbsp chocolate chips

Directions:

1 Turn on waffle maker to heat and oil it with cooking spray.
   Mix all dry components in a bowl.

2 Add egg and mix well.

3 Add cheese and stir again.

4 Spoon batter into waffle maker and close. Cook for 5
   minutes, until done. Top with whipping cream, cherries, and
   chocolate chips.

Nutrition Value per Servings:

Carbs - 6 G Fat - 1 G Protein - 1 G Calories – 130

Banana Nut Chaffle

Servings: 1

Prep time: 15 min.Cook time: 10 min.

Ingredients:

1 egg

1 Tbsp cream cheese, softened and room temp

1 Tbsp sugar-free cheesecake pudding ½ cup mozzarella cheese 1 Tbsp monk fruit confectioners sweetener ¼ tsp vanilla extract

¼ tsp banana extract toppings of choice

Directions:

1 Turn on waffle maker to heat and oil it with cooking spray. Beat egg in a small bowl.

2 Add remaining ingredients and mix until well incorporated.

3 Add one half of the batter to waffle maker and cook for 4 minutes, until golden brown. Remove chaffle and add the other half of the batter.

4 Top with your optional toppings and serve warm! Nutrition Value per Servings:

Carbs - 2 G Fat - 7 G Protein - 8 G Calories – 119

Belgium Chaffles

Servings: 1

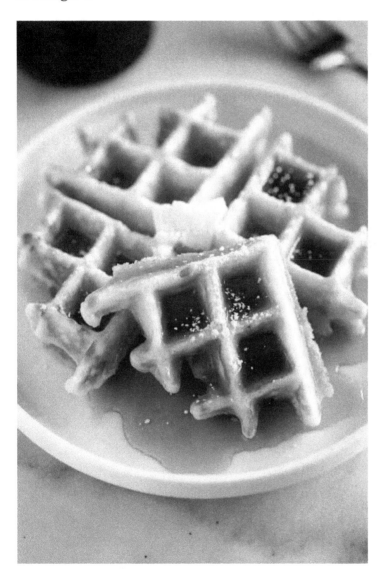

Prep time: 5 min. Cook time: 6 min. **Ingredients:**

2 eggs

1 cup Reduced-fat Cheddar cheese, shredded

Directions:

1 Turn on waffle maker to heat and oil it with cooking spray.

2 Whisk eggs in a bowl, add cheese. Stir until well-combined.

3 Pour mixture into waffle maker and cook for 6 minutes until done. Let it cool a little to crisp before serving.

Nutrition Value per Servings:

Carbs - 2 G Fat - 33 G Protein - 44 G Calories – 460

Bacon Chaffles

Servings: 2

Prep time: 5 min. Cook time: 5 min. **Ingredients:**

2 eggs

½ cup cheddar cheese

½ cup mozzarella cheese

¼ tsp baking powder

½ Tbsp almond flour

1 Tbsp butter, for waffle maker FOR THE FILLING:

¼ cup bacon, chopped

2 Tbsp green onions, chopped

Directions:

1 Turn on waffle maker to heat and oil it with cooking spray.

2 Add eggs, mozzarella, cheddar, almond flour, and baking powder to a blender and pulse 10 times, so cheese is still chunky.

3 Add bacon and green onions. Pulse 2-3 times to combine.

4 Add one half of the batter to the waffle maker and cook for 3 minutes, until golden brown.

5 Repeat with remaining batter. Add your toppings and serve ot. Nutrition Value per Servings:

Carbs - 3 G Fat - 38 G Protein - 23 G Calories – 446

Chaffle Egg Sandwich

Servings: 2

Cooking Time: 10 Minutes

Ingredients:

2 minutesI keto chaffle 2 slice cheddar cheese 1 egg simple omelet **Directions:**

1. Prepare your oven on 4000 F.

2. Arrange egg omelet and cheese slice between chaffles.

3. Bake in the preheated oven for about 4-5 minutes until cheese is melted.

4. Once the cheese is melted, remove from the oven.

5. Serve and enjoy! Nutrition value per Servings:

Protein: 144 kcal Fat: 337 kcal Carbohydrates: 14 kcal

Chaffle Minutesi Sandwich

Servings: 2

Cooking Time: 10 Minutes

Ingredients:

1 large egg

1/8 cup almond flour 1/2 tsp. garlic powder 3/4 tsp. baking powder 1/2 cup shredded cheese <u>SANDWICH FILLING:</u>

2 slices deli ham 2 slices tomatoes

1 slice cheddar cheese

Directions:

1. Grease your square waffle maker and preheat it on medium heat.

2. Mix chaffle ingredients in a mixing bowl until well combined.

3. Pour batter intoa square waffle and make two chaffles.

4. Once chaffles are cooked, remove from the maker.

5. For a sandwich,arrange deli ham, tomato slice and cheddar cheese between two chaffles.

6. Cut sandwich from the center.

7. Serve and enjoy! Nutrition value per Servings:

Calories 208 Fat 13.5g Carbohydrate 0.7g Protein 8.2g Sugars 0.6g

Chaffle Cheese Sandwich

Servings: 1

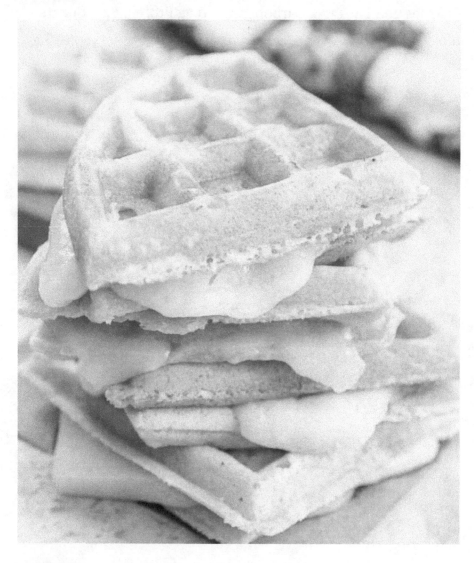

Cooking Time: 10 Minutes

Ingredients:

2 square keto chaffle 2 slice cheddar cheese

2 lettuce leaves

Directions:

1. Prepare your oven on 4000 F.

2. Arrange lettuce leave and cheese slice between chaffles.

3. Bake in the preheated oven for about 4-5 minutes until cheese is melted.

4. Once the cheese is melted, remove from the oven.

5. Serve and enjoy! Nutrition value per Servings:

Calories 208 Fat 13.5g Carbohydrate 0.7g Protein 8.2g Sugars 0.6g

Chicken Zinger Chaffle

Servings:2

Cooking Time: 15 Minutes

Ingredients:

1 chicken breast, cut into 2 pieces 1/2 cup coconut flour 1/4 cup finely grated Parmesan

1 tsp. paprika

1/2 tsp. garlic powder 1/2 tsp. onion powder 1 tsp. salt& pepper

1 egg beaten

Avocado oil for frying Lettuce leaves BBQ sauce

CHAFFLE Ingredients: 4 oz. cheese

2 whole eggs

2 oz. almond flour 1/4 cup almond flour 1 tsp baking powder

Directions:

1.   Mix chaffle ingredients in a bowl.

2.   Pour the chaffle batter in preheated greased square chaffle maker.

3.   Cook chaffles for about 2-minutes until cooked through.

4. Make square chaffles from this batter.

5. Meanwhile mix coconut flour, parmesan, paprika, garlic powder, onion powder salt and pepper in a bowl.

6. Dip chicken first in coconut flour mixture then in beaten egg.

7. Heat avocado oil in a skillet and cook chicken from both sides. until lightly brown and cooked

8. Set chicken zinger between two chaffles with lettuce and BBQ sauce.

9. Enjoy!

Nutrition value per Servings:

Calories 208 Fat 13.5g Carbohydrate 0.7g Protein 8.2g Sugars 0.6g

Double Chicken Chaffles

Servings:2

Cooking Time: 5 Minutes

Ingredients:

1/2 cup boil shredded chicken 1/4 cup cheddar cheese

1/8 cup parmesan cheese 1 egg

1 tsp. Italian seasoning

1/8 tsp. garlic powder 1 tsp. cream cheese **Directions:**

1. Preheat the Belgian waffle maker.

2. Mix in chaffle ingredients in a bowl and mix.

3. Sprinkle 1 tbsp. of cheese in a waffle maker and pour in chaffle batter.

4. Pour 1 tbsp. of cheese over batter and close the lid.

5. Cook chaffles for about 4 to minutes.

6. Serve with a chicken zinger and enjoy the double chicken flavor. Nutrition value per Servings:

Calories 208 Fat 13.5g Carbohydrate 0.7g Protein 8.2g Sugars 0.6g

Chaffles With Topping

Servings: 3

Cooking Time: 10 Minutes

Ingredients:

1 large egg

1 tbsp. almond flour

1 tbsp. full-fat Greek yogurt 1/8 tsp baking powder

1/4 cup shredded Swiss cheese TOPPING

4oz. grillprawns

4 oz. steamed cauliflower mash 1/2 zucchini sliced 3 lettuce leaves

1 tomato, sliced

1 tbsp. flax seeds

Directions:

1. Make 3 chaffles with the given chaffles ingredients.

2. For serving, arrange lettuce leaves on each chaffle.

3. Top with zucchini slice, grill prawns, cauliflower mash and a tomato slice.

4. Drizzle flax seeds on top.

5. Serve and enjoy! Nutrition value per Servings:

Calories 208 Fat 13.5g Carbohydrate 0.7g Protein 8.2g Sugars 0.6g

Chaffle With Cheese & Bacon

Servings:2

Cooking Time: 15 Minutes

ingredients:

1 egg

1/2 cup cheddar cheese, shredded 1 tbsp. parmesan cheese

3/4 tsp coconut flour 1/4 tsp baking powder

1/8 tsp Italian Seasoning pinch of salt

1/4 tsp garlic powder

FOR TOPPING

1 bacon sliced, cooked and chopped 1/2 cup mozzarella cheese, shredded

1/4 tsp parsley, chopped

Directions:

1. Preheat oven to 400 degrees.

2. Switch on your minutesi waffle maker and grease with cooking spray.

3. Mix chaffle ingredients in a mixing bowl until combined.

4. Spoon half of the batter in the center of the waffle maker and close the lid. Cook chaffles for about 3-minutes until cooked.

5. Carefully remove chaffles from the maker.

6. Arrange chaffles in a greased baking tray.

7. Top with mozzarella cheese, chopped bacon and parsley.

8. And bake in the oven for 4 -5 minutes.

9. Once the cheese is melted, remove from the oven.

10. Serve and enjoy! Nutrition value per Servings:

Calories 208 Fat 13.5g Carbohydrate 0.7g Protein 8.2g Sugars 0.6g

Grill Beefsteak And Chaffle

Servings: 1

Cooking Time: 10 Minutes

Ingredients:

1 beefsteak rib eye 1 tsp salt

1 tsp pepper

1 tbsp. lime juice 1 tsp garlic **Directions:**

1. Prepare your grill for direct heat.

2. Mix all spices and rub over beefsteak evenly.

3. Place the beef on the grill rack over medium heat.

4. Cover and cook steak for about6 to 8 minutes. Flip and cook for another 5 minutes until cooked through.

5. Serve with keto simple chaffle and enjoy! Nutrition value per Servings:

Calories 208 Fat 13.5g Carbohydrate 0.7g Protein 8.2g Sugars 0.6g

Cauliflower Chaffles And Tomatoes

Servings:2

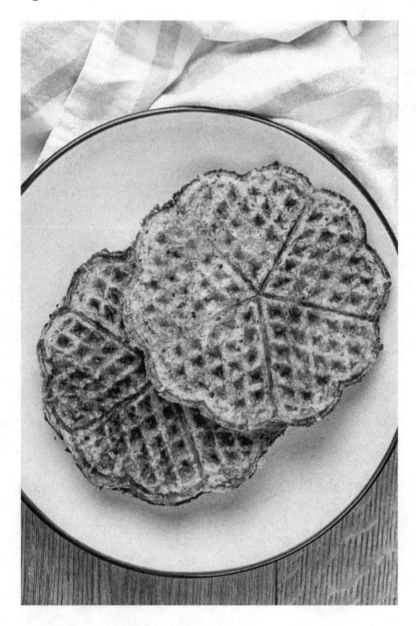

Cooking Time: 15 Minutes

Ingredients:

1/2 cup cauliflower 1/4 tsp. garlic powder 1/4 tsp. black pepper 1/4 tsp. Salt

1/2 cup shredded cheddar cheese 1 egg

FOR TOPPING

1 lettuce leave

1 tomato sliced

4 oz. cauliflower steamed, mashed 1 tsp sesame seeds

Directions:

1. Add all chaffle ingredients into a blender and mix well.

2. Sprinkle 1/8 shredded cheese on the waffle maker and pour cauliflower mixture in a preheated waffle maker and sprinkle the rest of the cheese over

it.

3. Cook chaffles for about 4-5 minutes until cooked

4. For serving, lay lettuce leaves over chaffle top with steamed cauliflower and tomato.

5. Drizzle sesame seeds on top.

6. Enjoy!

Nutrition value per Servings:

Calories 208 Fat 13.5g Carbohydrate 0.7g Protein 8.2g Sugars 0.6g

Layered Cheese Chaffles

Servings: 1

Cooking Time: 5 Minutes

Ingredients:

1 organic egg, beaten

1/3 cup Cheddar cheese, shredded

½ teaspoon ground flaxseed

¼ teaspoon organic baking powder

2 tablespoons Parmesan cheese, shredded

Directions:

1. Preheat a mini waffle iron and then grease it.

2. In a bowl, place all the ingredients except Parmesan and beat until well combined.

3. Place half the Parmesan cheese in the bottom of preheated waffle iron.

4. Place half of the egg mixture over cheese and top with the remaining Parmesan cheese.

5. Cook for about 3-minutes or until golden brown.

6. Serve warm.

Nutrition value per Servings:

Calories 208 Fat 13.5g Carbohydrate 0.7g Protein 8.2g Sugars 0.6g

Chaffles With Keto Ice Cream

Servings: 2

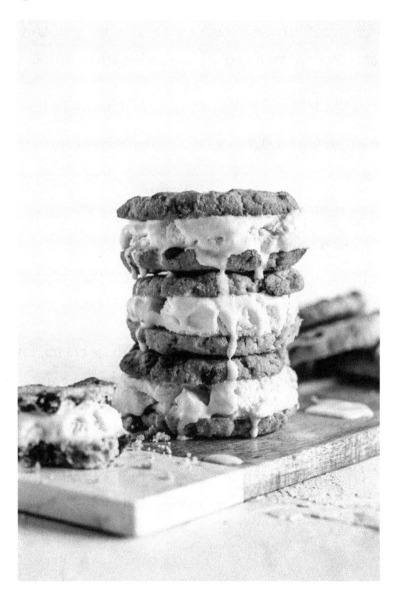

Cooking Time: 14 Minutes

Ingredients:

1 egg, beaten

½ cup finely grated mozzarella cheese ¼ cup almond flour 2 tbsp swerve confectioner's sugar 1/8 tsp xanthan gum Low-carb ice cream (flavor of your choice) for serving **Directions:**

1. Preheat the waffle iron.

2. In a medium bowl, mix all the ingredients except the ice cream.

3. Open the iron and add half of the mixture. Close and cook until crispy, 7 minutes.

4. Transfer the chaffle to a plate and make second one with the remaining batter.

5. On each chaffle, add a scoop of low carb ice cream, fold into half-moons and enjoy.

Nutrition value:

Calories 89 Fats 48g Carbs 1.67g Net Carbs 1.37g Protein 5.91g

Vanilla Mozzarella Chaffles

Servings: 2

Cooking Time: 12 Minutes

Ingredients:

1 organic egg, beaten

1 teaspoon organic vanilla extract 1 tablespoon almond flour

1 teaspoon organic baking powder Pinch of ground cinnamon 1 cup Mozzarella cheese, shredded

Directions:

1. Preheat a mini waffle iron and then grease it.

2. In a bowl, place the egg and vanilla extract and beat until well combined.

3. Add the flour, baking powder and cinnamon and mix well.

4. Add the Mozzarella cheese and stir to combine.

5. In a small bowl, place the egg and Mozzarella cheese and stir to combine.

6. Place half of the mixture into preheated waffle iron and cook for about 5- minutes or until golden brown.

7. Repeat with the remaining mixture.

8. Serve warm.

Nutrition value per Servings:

Calories 208 Fat 13.5g Carbohydrate 0.7g Protein 8.2g Sugars 0.6g

Bruschetta Chaffle

Servings: 2

Cooking Time: 5 Minutes

Ingredients:

2 basic chaffles

2 tablespoons sugar-free marinara sauce 2 tablespoons mozzarella, shredded

1 tablespoon olives, sliced 1 tomato sliced

1 tablespoon keto friendly pesto sauce Basil leaves

Directions:

1. Spread marinara sauce on each chaffle.

2. Spoon pesto and spread on top of the marinara sauce.

3. Top with the tomato, olives and mozzarella.

4. Bake in the oven for 3 minutes or until the cheese has melted.

5. Garnish with basil.

6. Serve and enjoy. Nutrition value:

Calories 208 Fat 13.5g Carbohydrate 0.7g Protein 8.2g Sugars
0.6g

Egg-Free Psyllium Husk Chaffles

Servings: 1

Cooking Time: 4 Minutes

Ingredients:

1 ounce Mozzarella cheese, shredded 1 tablespoon cream cheese, softened 1 tablespoon psyllium husk powder **Directions:**

1. Preheat a waffle iron and then grease it.

2. In a blender, place all ingredients and pulse until a slightly crumbly mixture forms.

3. Place the mixture into preheated waffle iron and cook for about 4 minutes or until golden brown.

4. Serve warm.

Nutrition value per Servings:

Calories 208 Fat 13.5g Carbohydrate 0.7g Protein 8.2g Sugars 0.6g

Mozzarella & Almond Flour Chaffles

Servings: 2

Cooking Time: 8 Minutes

Ingredients:

½ cup Mozzarella cheese, shredded 1 large organic egg

2 tablespoons blanched almond flour

¼ teaspoon organic baking powder

Directions:

1. Preheat a mini waffle iron and then grease it.

2. In a medium bowl, place all ingredients and with a fork, mix until well combined.

3. Place half of the mixture into preheated waffle iron and cook for about 4 minutes or until golden brown.

4. Repeat with the remaining mixture.

5. Serve warm.

Nutrition value per Servings:

Calories: 98 Fat: 7.1g Carbohydrates: 2.2g Sugar: 0.2g Protein: 7g

Pulled Pork Chaffle Sandwiches

Servings: 4

Cooking Time: 28 Minutes

Ingredients:

2 eggs, beaten

1 cup finely grated cheddar cheese ¼ tsp baking powder 2 cups cooked and shredded pork

1 tbsp sugar-free BBQ sauce 2 cups shredded coleslaw mix 2 tbsp apple cider vinegar

½ tsp salt

¼ cup ranch dressing

Directions:

1. Preheat the waffle iron.

2. In a medium bowl, mix the eggs, cheddar cheese, and baking powder.

3. Open the iron and add a quarter of the mixture. Close and cook until crispy, 7 minutes.

4. Transfer the chaffle to a plate and make 3 more chaffles in the same manner.

5. Meanwhile, in another medium bowl, mix the pulled pork with the BBQ sauce until well combined. Set aside.

6. Also, mix the coleslaw mix, apple cider vinegar, salt, and ranch dressing in another medium bowl.

7. When the chaffles are ready, on two pieces, divide the pork and then top with the ranch coleslaw. Cover with the remaining chaffles and insert mini skewers to secure the sandwiches.

8. Enjoy afterward. Nutrition value:

Calories 374 Fats 23.61g Carbs 8.2g Net Carbs 8.2g Protein 28.05g

Cheddar & Egg White Chaffles

Servings: 4

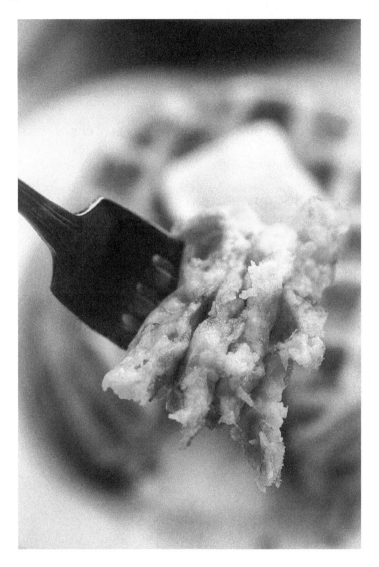

Cooking Time: 12 Minutes

Ingredients:

2 egg whites

1 cup Cheddar cheese, shredded

Directions:

1. Preheat a mini waffle iron and then grease it.

2. In a small bowl, place the egg whites and cheese and stir to combine.

3. Place ¼ of the mixture into preheated waffle iron and cook for about 4 minutes or until golden brown.

4. Repeat with the remaining mixture.

5. Serve warm.

Nutrition value per Servings:

Calories: 122 Fat: 9.4g Carbohydrates: 0.5g Sugar: 0.3g Protein: 8.8g

Spicy Shrimp And Chaffles

Servings: 4

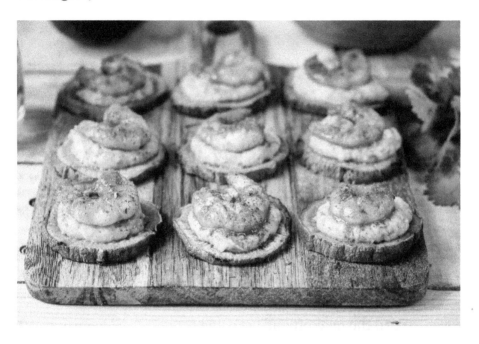

Cooking Time: 31 Minutes

Ingredients:

For the shrimp:

1 tbsp olive oil

1lb jumbo shrimp, peeled

1tbsp Creole seasoning

Salt to taste

1 tbsp hot sauce 3 tbsp butter

2 tbsp chopped fresh scallions to garnish For the chaffles: 2 eggs, beaten

1 cup finely grated Monterey Jack cheese

Directions:

1. For the shrimp:

2. Heat the olive oil in a medium skillet over medium heat.

3. Season the shrimp with the Creole seasoning and salt. Cook in the oil until pink and opaque on both sides, 2 minutes.

4. Pour in the hot sauce and butter. Mix well until the shrimp is adequately coated in the sauce, 1 minute.

5. Turn the heat off and set aside.

6. For the chaffles:

7. Preheat the waffle iron.

8. In a medium bowl, mix the eggs and Monterey Jack cheese.

9. Open the iron and add a quarter of the mixture. Close and cook until crispy, 7 minutes.

10. Transfer the chaffle to a plate and make 3 more chaffles in the same manner.

11. Cut the chaffles into quarters and place on a plate.

12. Top with the shrimp and garnish with the scallions.

13. Serve warm. Nutrition value:

Calories 342 Fats 19.75g Carbs 2.8g Net Carbs 2.3g Protein 36.01g

Creamy Chicken Chaffle Sandwich

Servings: 2

Cooking Time: 10 Minutes

Ingredients:

Cooking spray

1 cup chicken breast fillet, cubed Salt and pepper to taste

¼ cup all-purpose cream 4 garlic chaffles

Parsley, chopped

Directions:

1. Spray your pan with oil.

2. Put it over medium heat.

3. Add the chicken fillet cubes.

4. Season with salt and pepper.

5. Reduce heat and add the cream.

6. Spread chicken mixture on top of the chaffle.

7. Garnish with parsley and top with another chaffle.
   Nutrition value:

Calories 273 Fat 34g Saturated Fat 4.1g Carbohydrate 22. Sugars 3.2g Protein 17.5g

Chaffle Cannoli

Servings: 4

Cooking Time: 28 Minutes

Ingredients: For the chaffles: 1 large egg

1 egg yolk

3 tbsp butter, melted

1 tbso swerve confectioner's

1 cup finely grated Parmesan cheese

2 tbsp finely grated mozzarella cheese For the cannoli filling:

½ cup ricotta cheese

2 tbsp swerve confectioner's sugar 1 tsp vanilla extract

2 tbsp unsweetened chocolate chips for garnishing

Directions:

1. Preheat the waffle iron.

2. Meanwhile, in a medium bowl, mix all the ingredients for the chaffles.

3. Open the iron, pour in a quarter of the mixture, cover, and cook until crispy, 7 minutes.

4. Remove the chaffle onto a plate and make 3 more with the remaining batter.

5. Meanwhile, for the cannoli filling:

6. Beat the ricotta cheese and swerve confectioner's sugar until smooth. Mix in the vanilla.

7. On each chaffle, spread some of the filling and wrap over.

8. Garnish the creamy ends with some chocolate chips.

9. Serve immediately. Nutrition value:

Calories 308 Fats 25.05g Carbs 5.17g Net Carbs 5.17g Protein 15.18g

Strawberry Shortcake Chaffle Bowls

Servings: 4

Cooking Time: 28 Minutes

Ingredients:

1 egg, beaten

½ cup finely grated mozzarella cheese 1 tbsp almond flour

¼ tsp baking powder

2 drops cake batter extract

1 cup cream cheese, softened 1 cup fresh strawberries, sliced 1 tbsp sugar-free maple syrup **Directions:**

1. Preheat a waffle bowl maker and grease lightly with cooking spray.

2. Meanwhile, in a medium bowl, whisk all the ingredients except the cream cheese and strawberries.

3. Open the iron, pour in half of the mixture, cover, and cook until crispy, 6 to 7 minutes.

4. Remove the chaffle bowl onto a plate and set aside.

5. Make a second chaffle bowl with the remaining batter.

6. To serve, divide the cream cheese into the chaffle bowls and top with the strawberries.

7. Drizzle the filling with the maple syrup and serve.
   Nutrition value:

Calories 235 Fats 20.62g Carbs 5.9g Net Carbs 5g Protein 7.51g

Chocolate Melt Chaffles

Servings: 4

Cooking Time: 36 Minutes

Ingredients:

For the chaffles:

2 eggs, beaten

¼ cup finely grated Gruyere cheese 2 tbsp heavy cream

1 tbsp coconut flour

2 tbsp cream cheese, softened

3 tbsp unsweetened cocoa powder 2 tsp vanilla extract

A pinch of salt

For the chocolate sauce:

1/3 cup + 1 tbsp heavy cream

1 ½ oz unsweetened baking chocolate, chopped 1 ½ tsp sugar-free maple syrup

1 ½ tsp vanilla extract

Directions:

1. For the chaffles:

2. Preheat the waffle iron.

3. In a medium bowl, mix all the ingredients for the chaffles.

4. Open the iron and add a quarter of the mixture. Close and cook until crispy, 7 minutes. 5. Transfer the chaffle to a plate and make 3 more with the remaining batter.

6. For the chocolate sauce:

7. Pour the heavy cream into saucepan and simmer over low heat, 3 minutes.

8. Turn the heat off and add the chocolate. Allow melting for a few minutes and stir until fully melted, 5 minutes.

9. Mix in the maple syrup and vanilla extract.

10. Assemble the chaffles in layers with the chocolate sauce sandwiched

between each layer.

11. Slice and serve immediately. Nutrition value:

Calories 172 Fats 13.57g Carbs 6.65g Net Carbs 3.65g Protein 5.76g

Pumpkin & Pecan Chaffle

Servings: 2

Cooking Time: 10 Minutes

Ingredients:

1 egg, beaten

½ cup mozzarella cheese, grated

½ teaspoon pumpkin spice

1 tablespoon pureed pumpkin 2 tablespoons almond flour

1 teaspoon sweetener

2 tablespoons pecans, chopped

Directions:

1. Turn on the waffle maker.

2. Beat the egg in a bowl.

3. Stir in the rest of the ingredients.

4. Pour half of the mixture into the device.

5. Seal the lid.

6. Cook for 5 minutes.

7. Remove the chaffle carefully.

8. Repeat the steps to make the second chaffle. Nutrition value:

Calories 210 Total Fat 17 g Carbohydrate 4.6 g Protein 11 g Total Sugars 2 g

Spicy Jalapeno & Bacon Chaffles

Servings:2

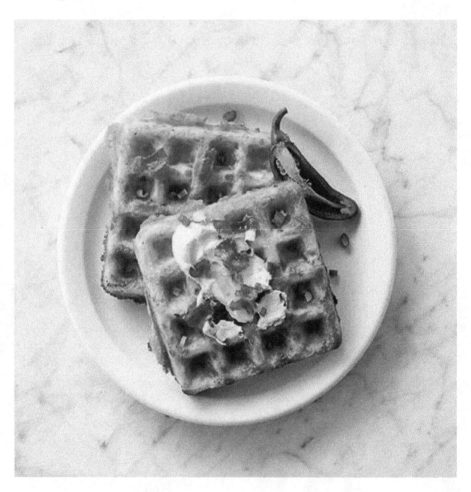

Cooking Time: 5 Minutes

Ingredients:

1 oz. cream cheese 1 large egg

1/2 cup cheddar cheese 2 tbsps. bacon bits

1/2 tbsp. jalapenos 1/4 tsp baking powder **Directions:**

1. Switch on your waffle maker.

2. Grease your waffle maker with cooking spray and let it heat up.

3. Mix egg and vanilla extract in a bowl first.

4. Add baking powder, jalapenos and bacon bites.

5. Add in cheese last and mix.

6. Pour the chaffles batter intothe maker and cook the chaffles for about 2-3 minutes.

7. Once chaffles are cooked, remove from the maker.

8. Serve hot and enjoy! Nutrition value per Servings:

Calories 172 Fats 13.57g Carbs 6.65g Net Carbs 3.65g Protein 5.76g

Zucchini Parmesan Chaffles

Servings: 2

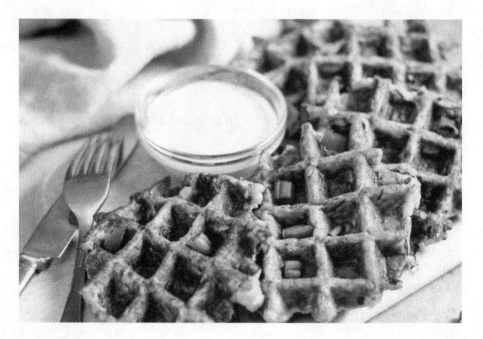

Cooking Time: 14 Minutes

Ingredients:

1 cup shredded zucchini 1 egg, beaten

½ cup finely grated Parmesan cheese

Salt and freshly ground black pepper to taste

Directions:

1. Preheat the waffle iron.

2. Put all the ingredients in a medium bowl and mix well.

3. Open the iron and add half of the mixture. Close and cook until crispy, 7 minutes.

4. Remove the chaffle onto a plate and make another with the remaining mixture.

5. Cut each chaffle into wedges and serve afterward. Nutrition value per Servings:

Calories 138 Fats 9.07g Carbs 3.81g Net Carbs 3.71g Protein 10.02g

Cheddar & Almond Flour Chaffles

Servings: 2

Cooking Time: 10 Minutes

Ingredients:

1 large organic egg, beaten

½ cup Cheddar cheese, shredded 2 tablespoons almond flour
Directions:

1. Preheat a mini waffle iron and then grease it.

2. In a bowl, place the egg, Cheddar cheese and almond flour and beat until well combined.

3. Place half of the mixture into preheated waffle iron and cook for about 5 minutes or until golden brown.

4. Repeat with the remaining mixture.

5. Serve warm.

Nutrition value per Servings:

Calories: 195 Fat: 15g Carbohydrates: 1.8g Sugar: 0.6g Protein: 10.2g

Simple& Beginner Chaffle

Servings:2

Cooking Time: 5 Minutes

Ingredients:

1 large egg

1/2 cup mozzarella cheese, shredded Cooking spray

Directions:

1. Switch on your waffle maker.

2. Beat the egg with a fork in a small mixing bowl.

3. Once the egg is beaten, add the mozzarella and mix well.

4. Spray the waffle makerwith cooking spray.

5. Pour the chaffles mixture in a preheated waffle maker and let it cook for about 2-3 minutes.

6. Once the chaffles are cooked, carefully remove them from the maker and cook the remaining batter.

7. Serve hot with coffee and enjoy! Nutrition value per Servings:

Protein: 36% 42 kcal Fat: 60% 71 kcal Carbohydrates: 4% 5 kcal

Asian Cauliflower Chaffles

Servings: 4

Cooking Time: 28 Minutes

Ingredients:

For the chaffles:

1 cup cauliflower rice, steamed 1 large egg, beaten

Salt and freshly ground black pepper to taste 1 cup finely grated Parmesan cheese

1 tsp sesame seeds

¼ cup chopped fresh scallions For the dipping sauce: 3 tbsp coconut aminos

1 ½ tbsp plain vinegar 1 tsp fresh ginger puree 1 tsp fresh garlic paste 3 tbsp sesame oil

1 tsp fish sauce

1 tsp red chili flakes

Directions:

1. Preheat the waffle iron.

2. In a medium bowl, mix the cauliflower rice, egg, salt, black pepper, and Parmesan cheese.

3. Open the iron and add a quarter of the mixture. Close and cook until crispy, 7 minutes.

4. Transfer the chaffle to a plate and make 3 more chaffles in the same manner.

5. Meanwhile, make the dipping sauce.

6. In a medium bowl, mix all the ingredients for the dipping sauce.

7. Plate the chaffles, garnish with the sesame seeds and scallions and serve with the dipping sauce.

Nutrition value:

Calories 231 Fats 188g Carbs 6.32g Net Carbs 5.42g Protein 9.66g

Sharp Cheddar Chaffles

Servings: 2

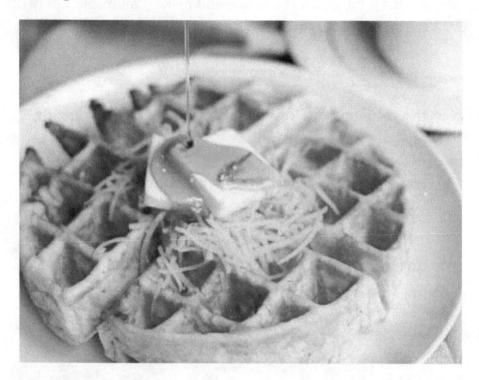

Cooking Time: 10 Minutes

Ingredients:

1 organic egg, beaten

½ cup sharp Cheddar cheese, shredded

Directions:

1. Preheat a mini waffle iron and then grease it.

2. In a small bowl, place the egg and cheese and stir to combine.

3. Place half of the mixture into preheated waffle iron and cook for about 5 minutes or until golden brown.

4. Repeat with the remaining mixture.

5. Serve warm.

Nutrition value per Servings:

Calories: 145 Fat: 11. Carbohydrates: 8.5g Protein: 9.8g

Egg-Free Almond Flour Chaffles

Servings: 2

Cooking Time: 10 Minutes

Ingredients:

2 tablespoons cream cheese, softened 1 cup mozzarella cheese, shredded

2 tablespoons almond flour

1 teaspoon organic baking powder

Directions:

1. Preheat a mini waffle iron and then grease it.

2. In a medium bowl, place all ingredients and with a fork, mix until well combined.

3. Place half of the mixture into preheated waffle iron and cook for about 4- 5 minutes or until golden brown.

4. Repeat with the remaining mixture.

5. Serve warm.

Nutrition value per Servings:

Calories: 77 Fat: 9.8g Carbohydrates: 3.2g Sugar: 0.3g Protein: 4.8g

Mozzarellas & Psyllium Husk Chaffles

Servings: 2

Cooking Time: 8 Minutes

Ingredients:

½ cup Mozzarella cheese, shredded 1 large organic egg, beaten

2 tablespoons blanched almond flour

½ teaspoon Psyllium husk powder

¼ teaspoon organic baking powder

Directions:

1. Preheat a mini waffle iron and then grease it.

2. In a bowl, place all the ingredients and beat until well combined.

3. Place half of the mixture into preheated waffle iron and cook for about 4 minutes or until golden brown.

4. Repeat with the remaining mixture.

5. Serve warm.

Nutrition value per Servings:

Calories: 101 Net Carb: 1. Fat: 7g Carbohydrates: 2.9g Sugar: 0.2g Protein: 6.7g

Pumpkin-Cinnamon Churro Sticks

Servings: 2

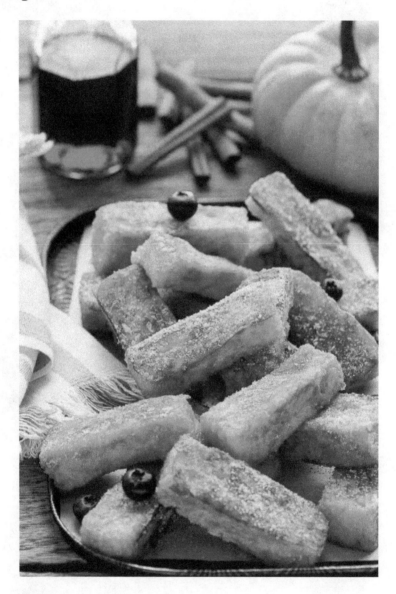

Cooking Time: 14 Minutes

Ingredients:

3 tbsp coconut flour

¼ cup pumpkin puree 1 egg, beaten

½ cup finely grated mozzarella cheese

2 tbsp sugar-free maple syrup + more for serving 1 tsp baking powder

1 tsp vanilla extract

½ tsp pumpkin spice seasoning 1/8 tsp salt

1 tbsp cinnamon powder

Directions:

1. Preheat the waffle iron.

2. Mix all the ingredients in a medium bowl until well combined.

3. Open the iron and add half of the mixture. Close and cook until golden brown and crispy, 7 minutes.

4. Remove the chaffle onto a plate and make 1 more with the remaining batter.

5. Cut each chaffle into sticks, drizzle the top with more maple syrup and serve after.

Nutrition value per Servings:

Calories 219 Fats 9.72g Carbs 8.g Net Carbs 4.34g Protein
25.27g

Chicken Jalapeño Chaffles

Servings: 2

Cooking Time: 14 Minutes

Ingredients:

1/8 cup finely grated Parmesan cheese

¼ cup finely grated cheddar cheese 1 egg, beaten

½ cup cooked chicken breasts, diced

1 small jalapeño pepper, deseeded and minced 1/8 tsp garlic powder 1/8 tsp onion powder

1 tsp cream cheese, softened

Directions:

1. Preheat the waffle iron.

2. In a medium bowl, mix all the ingredients until adequately combined.

3. Open the iron and add half of the mixture. Close and cook until crispy, 7 minutes.

4. Transfer the chaffle to a plate and make a second chaffle in the same manner.

5. Allow cooling and serve afterward. Nutrition value:

Calories 201 Fats 11.49g Carbs 3.7 Net Carbs 3.36g Protein 20.11g

Chocolate & Almond Chaffle

Servings: 3

Cooking Time: 12 Minutes

Ingredients:

1 egg

¼ cup mozzarella cheese, shredded 1 oz. cream cheese

2 teaspoons sweetener

1 teaspoon vanilla

2 tablespoons cocoa powder 1 teaspoon baking powder

2 tablespoons almonds, chopped

4 tablespoons almond flour

Directions:

1. Blend all the ingredients in a bowl while the waffle maker is preheating.

2. Pour some of the mixture into the waffle maker.

3. Close and cook for 4 minutes.

4. Transfer the chaffle to a plate. Let cool for 2 minutes.

5. Repeat steps using the remaining mixture. Nutrition value:

Calories 219 Total Fat 13.1g Carbohydrate 9.1g Fiber 3.8g
Protein 7.8g Sugars 0.8g

Keto Chocolate Fudge Chaffle

Servings: 2

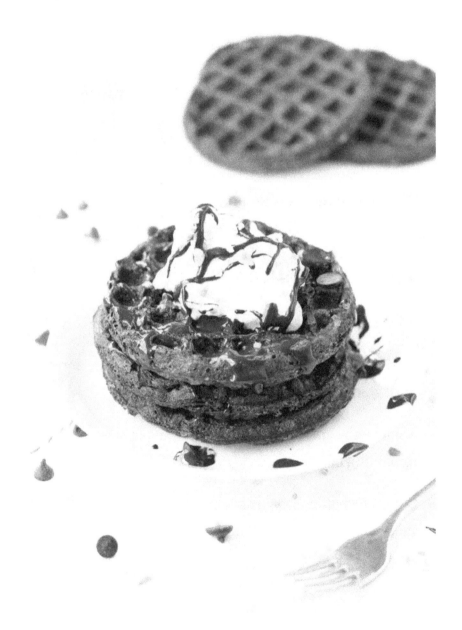

Cooking Time: 14 Minutes

Ingredients:

1 egg, beaten

¼ cup finely grated Gruyere cheese

2 tbsp unsweetened cocoa powder ¼ tsp baking powder

¼ tsp vanilla extract 2 tbsp erythritol

1 tsp almond flour

1 tsp heavy whipping cream A pinch of salt

Directions:

1. Preheat the waffle iron.

2. Add all the ingredients to a medium bowl and mix well.

3. Open the iron and add half of the mixture. Close and cook until golden brown and crispy, 7 minutes.

4. Remove the chaffle onto a plate and make another with the remaining batter.

5. Cut each chaffle into wedges and serve after. Nutrition value per Servings:

Calories 173 Fats 13.08g Carbs 3.98g Net Carbs 2.28g Protein 12.27g

Broccoli & Cheese Chaffle

Servings: 2

Cooking Time: 8 Minutes

Ingredients:

¼ cup broccoli florets 1 egg, beaten

1 tablespoon almond flour

¼ teaspoon garlic powder

½ cup cheddar cheese

Directions:

1. Preheat your waffle maker.

2. Add the broccoli to the food processor.

3. Pulse until chopped.

4. Add to a bowl.

5. Stir in the egg and the rest of the ingredients.

6. Mix well.

7. Pour half of the batter to the waffle maker.

8. Cover and cook for 4 minutes.

9. Repeat procedure to make the next chaffle. Nutrition value:

Calories 170 Total Fat 13 g Carbohydrate 2 g Protein 11 g Total
Sugars 1 g

Chaffled Brownie Sundae

Servings: 4

Cooking Time: 30 Minutes

Ingredients:

For the chaffles:

2 eggs, beaten

1 tbsp unsweetened cocoa powder 1 tbsp erythritol

1 cup finely grated mozzarella cheese For the topping: 3 tbsp unsweetened chocolate, chopped

3 tbsp unsalted butter

½ cup swerve sugar

Low-carb ice cream for topping 1 cup whipped cream for topping 3 tbsp sugar-free caramel sauce **Directions:**

1. For the chaffles:

2. Preheat the waffle iron.

3. Meanwhile, in a medium bowl, mix all the ingredients for the chaffles.

4. Open the iron, pour in a quarter of the mixture, cover, and cook until crispy, 7 minutes.

5. Remove the chaffle onto a plate and make 3 more with the remaining batter.

6. Plate and set aside.

7. For the topping:

8. Meanwhile, melt the chocolate and butter in a medium saucepan with occasional stirring, 2 minutes.

9. To Servings:

10. Divide the chaffles into wedges and top with the ice cream, whipped cream, and swirl the chocolate sauce and caramel sauce on top.

11. Serve immediately. Nutrition value:

Calories 165 Fats 11.39g Carbs 3.81g Net Carbs 2.91g Protein 79g

Cream Cheese Chaffle

Servings: 2

Cooking Time: 8 Minutes

Ingredients:

1 egg, beaten

1 oz. cream cheese

½ teaspoon vanilla

4 teaspoons sweetener

¼ teaspoon baking powder Cream cheese

Directions:

1. Preheat your waffle maker.

2. Add all the ingredients in a bowl.

3. Mix well.

4. Pour half of the batter into the waffle maker.

5. Seal the device.

6. Cook for 4 minutes.

7. Remove the chaffle from the waffle maker.

8. Make the second one using the same steps.

9. Spread remaining cream cheese on top before serving.
   Nutrition value:

Calories 169 Total Fat 14.3g Carbohydrate 4g Fiber 4g Protein 7.7g Sugars 0.7g

Beef And Tomato Chaffle

Servings:4

Cooking Time:15 Minutes

Ingredients:

Batter 4 eggs

¼ cup cream cheese

1 cup grated mozzarella cheese Salt and pepper to taste

¼ cup almond flour

1 teaspoon freshly chopped dill Beef

1 pound beef loin

Salt and pepper to taste

1 tablespoon balsamic vinegar 2 tablespoons olive oil

1 teaspoon freshly chopped rosemary

2 tablespoons cooking spray to brush the waffle maker 4 tomato slices for serving

Directions:

1.   Preheat the waffle maker.

2. Add the eggs, cream cheese, grated mozzarella cheese, salt and pepper, almond flour and freshly chopped dill to a bowl.

3. Mix until combined and batter forms.

4. Brush the heated waffle maker with cooking spray and add a few tablespoons of the batter.

5. Close the lid and cook for about 8-10 minutes depending on your waffle maker.

6. Meanwhile, heat the olive oil in a nonstick frying pan and season the beef loin with salt and pepper and freshly chopped rosemary.

7. Cook the beef on each side for about 5 minutes and drizzle with some balsamic vinegar. 8. Serve each chaffle with a slice of tomato and cooked beef loin slices.

Nutrition value per Servings:

Calories 4, fat 35.8 g, carbs 3.3 g, sugar 0.8 g, Protein 40.3 g

Classic Ground Pork Chaffle

Servings:4

Cooking Time:15 Minutes

Ingredients:

½ pound ground pork 3 eggs

½ cup grated mozzarella cheese Salt and pepper to taste 1 clove garlic, minced

1 teaspoon dried oregano

2 tablespoons butter to brush the waffle maker

2 tablespoons freshly chopped parsley for garnish

Directions:

1. Preheat the waffle maker.

2. Add the ground pork, eggs, mozzarella cheese, salt and pepper, minced garlic and dried oregano to a bowl.

3. Mix until combined.

4. Brush the heated waffle maker with butter and add a few tablespoons of the batter.

5. Close the lid and cook for about 7-8 minutes depending on your waffle maker.

6. Serve with freshly chopped parsley. Nutrition value per Servings:

Calories 192, fat 11.g, carbs 1 g, sugar 0.3 g, Protein 20.2 g

Beef Chaffle Taco

Servings:4

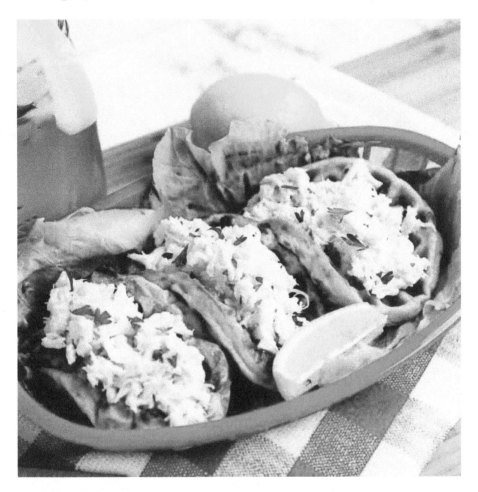

Cooking Time:15 Minutes

Ingredients:

Batter 4 eggs

1 cups grated cheddar cheese ¼ cup heavy cream Salt and pepper to taste

¼ cup almond flour

2 teaspoons baking powder Beef

2 tablespoons butter

½ onion, diced

1 pound ground beef Salt and pepper to taste

1 teaspoon dried oregano

1 tablespoon sugar-free ketchup

2 tablespoons cooking spray to brush the waffle maker 2 tablespoons freshly chopped parsley

Directions:

1. Preheat the waffle maker.

2. Add the eggs, grated cheddar cheese, heavy cream, salt and pepper, almond flour and baking powder to a bowl.

3. Brush the heated waffle maker with cooking spray and add a few tablespoons of the batter.

4. Close the lid and cook for about 5-7 minutes depending on your waffle maker.

5. Once the chaffle is ready, place it in a napkin holder to harden into the shape of a taco as it cools.

6. Meanwhile, melt and heat the butter in a nonstick frying pan and start cooking the diced onion.

7. Once the onion is tender, add the ground beef. Season with salt and pepper and dried oregano and stir in the sugar-free ketchup.

8. Cook for about 7 minutes.

9. Serve the cooked ground meat in each taco chaffle sprinkled with some freshly chopped parsley.

Nutrition value per Servings:

Calories 719, fat 51.7 g, carbs 7.3 g, sugar 1.3 g, Protein 56.1 g

Turkey Chaffle Sandwich

Servings:4

Cooking Time:15 Minutes

Ingredients:

Batter 4 eggs

¼ cup cream cheese

1 cup grated mozzarella cheese Salt and pepper to taste 1
teaspoon dried dill

½ teaspoon onion powder

½ teaspoon garlic powder Juicy chicken

2 tablespoons butter

1 pound chicken breast Salt and pepper to taste

1 teaspoon dried dill

2 tablespoons heavy cream

2 tablespoons butter to brush the waffle maker 4 lettuce leaves
to garnish the sandwich

4 tomato slices to garnish the sandwich

Directions:

1. Preheat the waffle maker.

2. Add the eggs, cream cheese, mozzarella cheese, salt and pepper, dried dill, onion powder and garlic powder to a bowl.

3. Mix everything with a fork just until batter forms.

4. Brush the heated waffle maker with butter and add a few tablespoons of the batter.

5. Close the lid and cook for about 7 minutes depending on your waffle maker.

6. Meanwhile, heat some butter in a nonstick pan.

7. Season the chicken with salt and pepper and sprinkle with dried dill. Pour the heavy cream on top.

8. Cook the chicken slices for about 10 minutes or until golden brown.

9. Cut each chaffle in half.

10. On one half add a lettuce leaf, tomato slice, and chicken slice. Cover with the other chaffle half to make a sandwich.

11. Serve and enjoy. Nutrition value per Servings:

Calories 381, fat 26.3 g, carbs 2.5 g, sugar 1 g, Protein 32.9 g

Bbq Sauce Pork Chaffle

Servings:4

Cooking Time:15 Minutes

Ingredients:

½ pound ground pork 3 eggs

1 cup grated mozzarella cheese Salt and pepper to taste 1 clove garlic, minced

1 teaspoon dried rosemary

3 tablespoons sugar-free BBQ sauce

2 tablespoons butter to brush the waffle maker ½ pound pork rinds for serving

¼ cup sugar-free BBQ sauce for serving

Directions:

1. Preheat the waffle maker.

2. Add the ground pork, eggs, mozzarella, salt and pepper, minced garlic, dried rosemary, and BBQ sauce to a bowl.

3. Mix until combined.

4. Brush the heated waffle maker with butter and add a few tablespoons of the batter.

5. Close the lid and cook for about 7-8 minutes depending on your waffle maker.

6. Serve each chaffle with some pork rinds and a tablespoon of BBQ sauce. Nutrition value per Servings:

Calories 350, fat 21.1 g, carbs 2.g, sugar 0.3 g, Protein 36.9 g

Simple Chaffles Without Maker

Servings:2

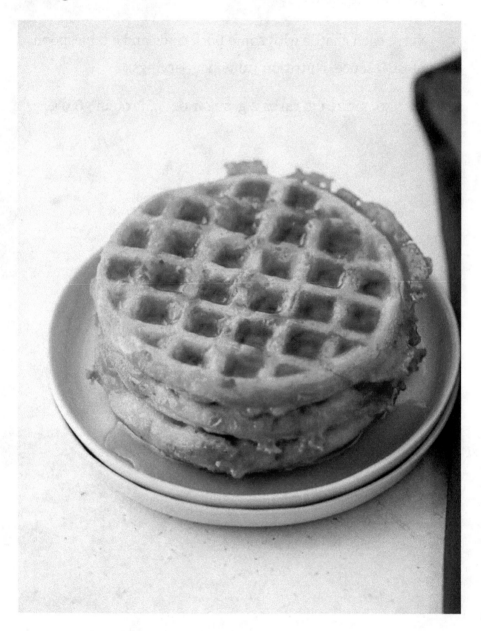

Cooking Time:5minutes

Ingredients:

1 tbsp. chia seeds 1 egg

1/2 cup cheddar cheese pinch of salt

1 tbsp. avocado oil

Directions:

1.   Heat your nonstick pan over medium heat

2.   In a small bowl, mix chia seeds, salt, egg, and cheese

3.   Grease pan with avocado oil.

4.   Once the pan is hot, pour 2 tbsps. chaffle batter and cook for about 1-2 minutes.

5.   Flip and cook for another 1-2 minutes.

6.   Once chaffle is brown remove from pan.

7.   Serve with berries on top and enjoy. Nutrition value per **Servings**:

Calories 132 Fat 5.5g Carbohydrate 1.6g Protein 6.4g Sugars 0.6g

Heart Shape Chaffles

Servings:2

Cooking Time:5 Minutes

Ingredients:

1 egg

1 cup mozzarella cheese 1 tsp baking powder

¼ cup almond flour 1 tbsp. coconut oil

Directions:

1.   Heat your nonstick pan over medium heat.

2.   Mix all ingredients in a bowl.

3.   Grease pan with avocado oil and place a heart shape cookie cutter over the pan.

4.   Once the pan is hot, pour the batter equally in 2 cutters.

5.   Cook for another 1-2 minutes.

6.   Once chaffle is set, remove the cutter, flip and cook for another 1-2 minutes.

7.   Once chaffles are brown, remove from the pan.

8.   Serve hot and enjoy! Nutrition value per Servings:

Calories 128 Fat 10.5g Carbohydrate 1.6g Protein 7.4g Sugars 0.6g

Bacon Chaffles With Herb Dip

Servings: 2

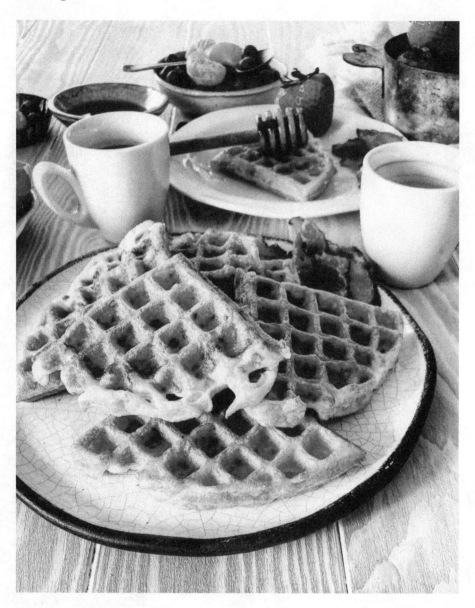

Cooking Time: 10 Minutes

Ingredients:

Chaffles

1 organic egg, beaten

½ cup Swiss/Gruyere cheese blend, shredded 2 tablespoons cooked bacon pieces

1 tablespoon jalapeño pepper, chopped Dip

¼ cup heavy cream

¼ teaspoon fresh dill, minced Pinch of ground black pepper

Directions:

1.   Preheat a mini waffle iron and then grease it.

2.   For chaffles: In a medium bowl, put all ingredients and mix well.

3.   Place half of the mixture into preheated waffle iron and cook for about 5 minutes.

4.   Repeat with the remaining mixture.

5.   Meanwhile, for dip: in a bowl, mix the cream and stevia.

6.   Serve warm chaffles alongside the dip. Nutrition value:

Calories 210 Fat 13 g Carbs 2.3 g Fiber 0.1 g Sugar 0.7 g Protein 11.9 g

Lobster Chaffle

Servings: 2

Cooking Time: 8 Minutes

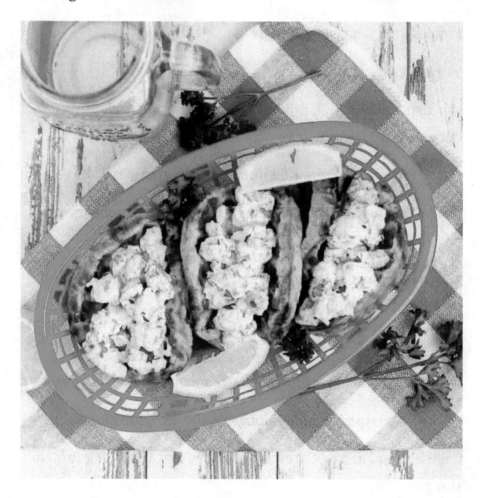

Ingredients:

1 egg (beaten)

½ cup shredded mozzarella cheese ¼ tsp garlic powder

¼ tsp onion powder

1/8 tsp Italian seasoning Lobster Filling:

½ cup lobster tails (defrosted) 1 tbsp mayonnaise

1 tsp dried basil 1 tsp lemon juice

1 tbsp chopped green onion

Directions:

1.   Plug the waffle maker to preheat it and spray it with a non-stick cooking spray.

2.   In a mixing bowl, combine the mozzarella, Italian seasoning, garlic and onion powder. Add the egg and mix until the ingredients are well combined.

3.   Pour an appropriate amount of the batter into the waffle maker and spread out the batter to cover all the holes on the waffle maker.

4.   Close the waffle maker and cook for about minutes or according to your waffle maker's settings.

5.   After the cooking cycle, use a plastic or silicone utensil to remove and transfer the chaffle to a wire rack to cool.

6.   Repeat step 3 to 5 until you have cooked all the batter into chaffles.

7.   For the filling, put the lobster tail in a mixing bowl and add the

mayonnaise, basil and lemon juice.

Toss until the ingredients are well combine.

8.   Fill the chaffles with the lobster mixture and garnish with chopped green onion.

9.   Serve and enjoy. Nutrition value per Servings:

Calories 168 Fat 15.5g Carbohydrate 1.6g Protein 5.4g Sugars 0.6g

9 781801 457422